HIGH OFF LIFE
The Turning Point:
12 Steps to Spiritual Freedom

High Off Life
The Turning Point:

12 Steps to Spiritual Freedom

Written by Lewis Burt

This book may be purchased in bulk for educational, business, or sales promotional use.

©2024 by Words of Wisdom Publishing. Published in Pittsburgh, PA.

Editor: *Stacey M. Robinson / KYA Publishing Canada*

Cover / Page Design by *Ashley Mae Pancho*

eBook Design by: *Osamudiamenabdul*

Contributions by *ElevatedWaves Publishing Corp.*

ISBN (Paperback): 979-8-9857424-6-6

ISBN (E-book): 979-8-9857424-7-3

Library of Congress Control Number (LCCN): 2024904338

Follow *Lewis Burt* **on social media:**

Twitter/X: @RealMrBurt

Instagram: @RealMrBurt

Facebook: @RealMrBurt

TABLE OF CONTENTS

TABLE OF CONTENTS

 DEDICATION

This book is dedicated to everyone who has experienced, those who are currently experiencing, and those who will experience some form of adversity in their lifetime.

Remember that you are resilient; your life has value and purpose regardless of what you may be experiencing at the moment. Please remain hopeful and remember that you are loved.

 ACKNOWLEDGMENTS

First and foremost, I must acknowledge God for using me as a vessel. Thank you, Lord, for opening my spiritual eyes and ears. Because of you, I feel purposeful.

Secondly, I would like to thank Derek Carlton and Bryan Janes for giving me motivation to put my pen to paper and write my story.

Lastly, I would like to thank my mother for always being my rock. Thank you!

 # ABOUT THE AUTHOR

Born and raised in Pittsburgh, Pennsylvania, Lewis Burt believes that a power greater than himself can restore him back to sanity.

High Of Life, The Turning Point: 12 Steps to Spiritual Freedom is a mirror into the heart and soul of Lewis—reflecting love, defeat, pain, maturity, and hope.

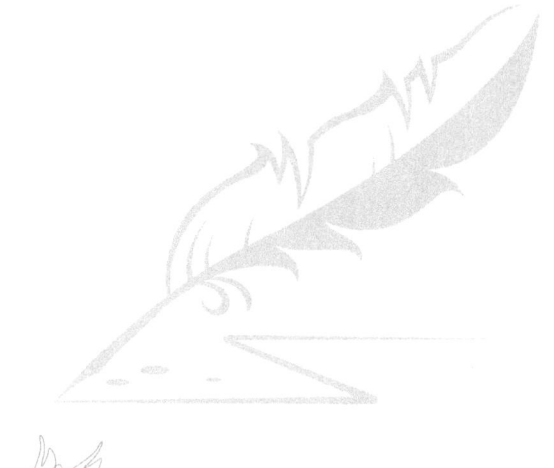

PREFACE

I have found an innovative way to not only tell my story *High Off Life, The Turning Point: 12 Steps to Spiritual Freedom*, but also to offer my story as a guide to help readers overcome adversity through faith and spiritual growth. I know what I experienced is much bigger than me, so I am compelled to share the lessons I learned throughout the most painful moments of my life. You will find that each entry in this book offers a title, poem, personal story, and path to spiritual freedom.

— • • • —

(Proverbs 20:1)

Wine produces mockers;
alcohol leads to brawls.
Those led astray by drink cannot be wise.

— • • • —

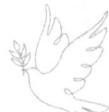

INTRODUCTION

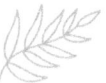

Drugs and alcohol had me shackled in chains. Even when the sun was shining bright, all I felt was the rain. The dark cloud of addiction—I was trapped in my pain. Drink after drink, but still feeling the same. I was digging my own grave, taking shot after shot. I felt my body shutting down, but my mind wouldn't let me stop. Am I an alcoholic? I asked myself in the mirror. I was holding a drink in my right hand, so the answer was clear. I'm disgusted in who I've become, and my heart is full of fear. My eyes are filled with tears because I know the end is near. How did I get here? I never thought this could be me. My tolerance keeps increasing. I'm trapped in my disease. Now I'm on my knees, asking God for help. I came to the realization that I couldn't do this by myself. God, please give me strength to overcome and conquer. Please loosen the Devil's grip and save me from this monster. God heard my cries, and I didn't have to wait any longer. God answered my prayers, and blessed me with a sponsor.

FROM ME TO YOU

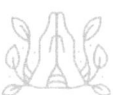

For years I was addicted to alcohol, and I always found an excuse to lie to myself. I would look directly in the mirror and act as if I didn't see an alcoholic staring right back at me. I convinced myself that I could never be labeled as someone who didn't have control over how much alcohol they consumed.

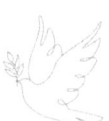

Living in denial and running from the truth led me down one of the darkest paths of my life.

Reality began to set in physically, mentally, emotionally, and spiritually. Physically, my body began to deteriorate right before my eyes. I could feel my liver beginning to fail, and I also lost a lot of weight because alcohol became more important to me than eating three square meals a day. I was mentally trapped inside the bottle, and my mind convinced me to ignore the physical abuse I was taking my body through from drinking too much alcohol.

All the drinking that I was doing to heal emotionally was only a temporary bandage. Every time I sobered up the pain was still there, and I was now nothing more than an alcoholic in pain. Spiritually, my faith remained strong, but the alcohol seemed to drift me further and further away from my connection with God.

Finding myself in the deepest, darkest pit of my life, I begged and pleaded to God to save me from the grips of alcoholism. Just as God has always done, he answered my prayers when I needed him the most. God gave me a ladder to climb out of the deep dark pit that I was trapped in.

God knew I was battling something that I couldn't defeat on my own. That's when God blessed me with a sponsor who immediately brought me out of the darkness and into the light.

The Turning Point

Nothing happens in God's world by mistake.

· · ·

(Galatians 6:10)

Therefore, as we have opportunity,

let us do good to all people,

especially to those who belong

to the family of believers.

· · ·

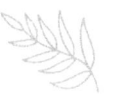 **MY SPONSOR**

I asked God to heal me from alcoholism,

and he didn't make me wait any longer.

In the blink of an eye, God blessed me with a sponsor.

His name is Derek Carlton, and he's a gift from God.

Doing God's will and servicing others is the title of his job.

It's rare to meet a person who puts others before themselves.

Before I met my sponsor, he extended his hand and offered help.

He introduced me to the big book and walked me through the steps.

He explained how alcoholism is an allergy, and I was able to reflect.

He helped me to internalize step three, and now I let it be Thy Will.

Now I see the part I played in my resentments,

and that really helped me to heal.

He taught me how to spot my character defects,

because they would be stuck with me for life.

Those defects could become principles if I learned to use them right.

He helped me to make amends,

and a weight was lifted off my shoulders.

My resentments were killing me, and my heart was getting colder.

Now I check my inventory daily, and practice humility and patience.

I stay connected to God through prayer and meditation.

This is a spiritual awakening. My eyes are open—now I see.

My will and my life are in the care of God

because he wants to build with me.

Now that I'm walking in my purpose, I'm ready to go conquer!

God saved my life when he blessed me with my sponsor.

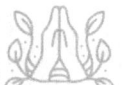 FROM ME TO YOU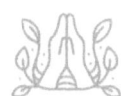

When I was a child and all the way until I stepped into adulthood, I would hear other people mention how they were going through a midlife crisis. I never could comprehend until I found myself in my deepest darkest moments.

My life came crashing down, and I became overwhelmed with pain and fear. I found myself stuck in isolation with nobody and nothing to turn to accept alcohol.

Alcohol became the crutch that I used to mask everything I was feeling. Alcohol became my temporary bandage, because it didn't stop the pain that consumed me on a daily basis. To be honest, alcohol made life more unbearable because I was now chained to a bottle that would eventually kill me.

What was even more devastating was that alcohol never helped cure any of the pain I was feeling!

One day in the midst of my alcohol addiction, I found myself on my knees begging for God's mercy. I prayed to God to rescue me from my addiction, and to relieve me of my current pain. Miraculously, God heard my cries and almost simultaneously blessed me with a sponsor who was able to pull me out of one of the darkest times of my life.

My sponsor had experienced everything I was experiencing in my midlife crisis. His transparency, wisdom, and knowledge made me curious to learn more about sobriety, and a new way of living.

I was then introduced to the Alcoholics Anonymous Big Book. Next, my Sponsor and I slowly but thoroughly began to work the twelve steps that The Big Book outlined. After step three, I was able to understand that nothing in my life was working in my favor because I was trying to control the events by doing things on my own will, and my own way.

When I finally submitted my will over to the care of God, my spiritual eyes were opened, and from that day forward I was able to see God's plan for my life.

The Turning Point

A good sponsor can guide you from the darkness to the light.

(Romans 5:3-5)

Not only so, but we also glory in our sufferings, because we know that suffering produces perseverance; perseverance, character; and character, hope. And hope does not put us to shame, because God's love has been poured out into our hearts through the Holy Spirit, who has been given to us.

THE FIRST STEP TO RECOVERY

My first step to recovery was being honest with myself.

God is the only one who can save me; I can't do this by myself.

If I let God guide my steps, I'll walk into my purpose.

No more drowning in my fears

because my head is above the surface.

If I continue to use my spiritual eyes, my vision will become clearer.

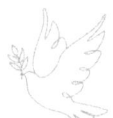

Then I can accept the reflection that I see

from the man in the mirror.

My confidence will rise, and my light will shine on others.

There's light at the end of our tunnels from one alcoholic to another.

To my sisters and my brothers: isolation can get lonely.

Step outside your comfort zones and fellowship

—let's share our testimonies.

There's beauty in the struggle, so don't be afraid to share your pain.

I have witnessed beautiful sunshine, but this is only after the rain.

I was running from my pain, until I learned to embrace it.

Don't try to drink away your trouble—learn how to face it.

Honestly is the key; there's no need to live a lie.

Where all God's children, like his angels, learn to fly.

Take your place in the sky, and let your purpose become your light.

When we submit our will to God, we shall learn his way of life.

I accepted my transformation, and now I'm finally feeling free.

Being honest with myself was the first step to my recovery.

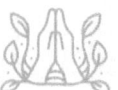 # FROM ME TO YOU

After I took my first step towards recovery by being honest with myself and admitting that I was an alcoholic, the turning point was then in motion. I finally accepted the fact that I couldn't drink like a normal person. Even more importantly, I accepted the fact that my next drink could lead me to the grave.

After I stopped lying to myself, I was able to open up to my sponsor and other alcoholics who were able to help me accept my truth by hearing their testimonies. Their testimonies exposed their pain, fear, and how they were unable to climb out of the bottle by themselves. This newfound fellowship brought me a sense of peace and belonging—I knew I was in connection with a group of unique individuals who all shared one thing in common: alcoholism.

Building with my sponsor and other alcoholics helped me to heal day by day. I found myself looking forward to going to AA meetings because in the fellowship I could hear God speaking directly to me through other people. This new experience in sobriety brought me a sense of peace and serenity. It was a new healing process that opened my mind and my heart.

With my feet planted solid on the road to recovery, it was the beginning of my rebirth. I became eager to learn more about AA, the twelve steps, and what The Big Book had to offer.

My name is Lewis Burt; I'm an alcoholic.

Today I'm able to walk in my truth.

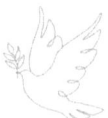

The Turning Point

Being honest with myself unlocked the door that led me to sobriety.

. . .

(Proverbs 1:7)

The fear of the Lord is
the beginning of knowledge,
but fools despise wisdom and instruction.

. . .

 # GIVING EVERYTHING TO GOD

I'm walking by faith; I'm not walking by sight.

God has a plan for us all, and the path is full of light.

My footsteps are guided by God almighty.

God wants to build with me, and I'm not going to fight it.

There's a power greater than myself

that can store me back to sanity.

If I submit my will to God, I don't have to try to manage this.

I don't want to damage this; I know my life is in God's hands.

I have control over nothing; everything is in God's plans.

Let it be Thy will—I learned that in Step Three.

God is driving and I'm the passenger

because He wants to build with me.

God has a purpose for my life that He's ready to uncover.

God wants to use me as His vessel, to shine my light on others.

This makes my heart smile, and I want to please God more!

God brought me back to sanity, and now I feel restored.

My faith has elevated because my life is in God's hands.

It was never my will, but always God's. Now I understand.

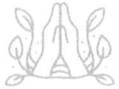 FROM ME TO YOU

One of the best decisions I've ever made was to turn my will and my life over to the care of God. After I finished Step Three in the AA Big Book, and after working with my sponsor, for the first time in my life I was able to understand God in a new light.

Throughout my life I always believed in God, and would say that my faith was pretty strong. I always believed that whatever happened to me—whether good or bad—was all a part of God's plan. For as long as I can remember, I would pray to God every morning, every night, and throughout the day.

This always brought me a sense of peace and serenity because I honestly believed that God would always hear my prayers.

After meeting my sponsor and being exposed to AA and The Big Book, my relationship with God became even more amazing. After I completed Step Three, something incredible happened: I became aware (for the first time in all my years of believing and trusting in God) that He wanted to be more involved in my life. I understood that God wanted me to fully turn my will and my life over to His care.

God wanted to take away my pain, my fears, my worries, and most importantly He wanted to build with me through His plans for my life. God wanted to help me become the best version of myself by simply letting it be Thy will.

This new understanding I had come to accept was that God was driving while I was in the passenger seat. This understanding instantly made life's ride a lot smoother. I came to accept that I could now let God drive me towards my purpose by buckling up my seatbelt and following His directions for my life through prayer and meditation.

I understand that for all who turn to Him, all will be well with them, here and hereafter.

The Turning Point

I began to live out my purpose when I let it be Thy will.

· · ·

(Romans 12:2)

Do not conform to the pattern of this world,
but be transformed by the renewing
of your mind. Then you will be able to test and
approve what God's will is—His good, pleasing,
and perfect will.

· · ·

FROM RESENTMENT TO PURITY

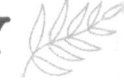

Resentment can be cancerous and detrimental to your health.

Resentment will eat away at your soul. I experienced it myself.

I was holding on to grudges and swallowing my anger.

I became a ticking time bomb, and that's a recipe for danger.

My heart was full of pain, and it was ready to explode.

I was dying on the inside, so I had to let it go.

When I learned to forgive, a weight was lifted off my shoulders.

I had to let it go because my heart was getting colder.

Now, I feel free from the anger and the pain.

I scrubbed resentment from my soul, and it didn't leave a stain.

I am no longer in pain, and I can step into my purpose.

Forgiveness has set me free, and I feel better on the surface.

Today when I feel resentful, I try to make amends.

That's the key to my serenity: I can't let resentment win!

Holding on to anger will begin to dim my light.

So I release it, and do Thy will, and move on with my life.

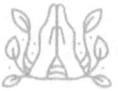 # FROM ME TO YOU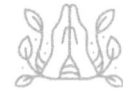

Do you know what resentment is? Resentment is the process of dwelling on a painful or upsetting situation to the point where it causes you anger and bitterness. Resentment can eat away at you and poison your heart against trusting others, feeling compassion, or being open to love in the future.

You can release resentment in five steps:

1. Acknowledge resentment. Since the process always starts with being honest with yourself, the first step to releasing resentment is to acknowledge that you feel resentful.

2. Identify where you have power.

3. Take action where you have power.

4. Release anything over which you don't have power.

5. Make gratitude a daily habit.

We often have resentment towards specific individuals, and issues arise because we haven't yet learned to address our resentment. Instead, we tend to hold it in and we end up paying the price for not releasing our pain.

Taking a searching and fearless moral inventory of ourselves is imperative. Learning to release anger, worry, self-pity, and depression by letting go of resentments can direct you to a life full of peace and serenity.

The Turning Point

When I realized that I played a part in all of my resentments, I was able to let go of a lot of anger I had stored up inside of me for years.

(Ephesians 4:22-24)

You were taught, with regard to your former way of life, to put off your old self, which is being corrupted by its deceitful desires; to be made new in the attitude of your minds; and to put on a new self, created to be like God in true righteousness and holiness.

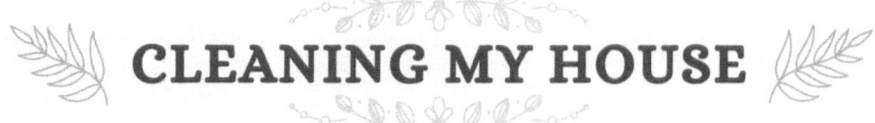

CLEANING MY HOUSE

A fearless moral inventory of myself is what I'm searching for.

If I let it be Thy will, then God will build with me for sure.

Discovering my liabilities was my blueprint through Step Four.

This is a lifetime practice so I can stay restored.

My willingness to take inventory has brought me light, and new confidence.

The tools that keep me grounded are God, and great sponsorship.

Self-justification is very dangerous for my health.

I refuse to make excuses to feel good about myself.

It's time I dust my shelves; I think I'll scrub my bathroom too!

I'm cleaning my house because I want to. Nobody asked me to.
A clean home is a happy home—that's the moral of this story.
It's time for me to vacuum my misguided inventory.

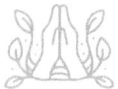 # FROM ME TO YOU

By the time I started doing my fourth step in AA, I was starting to actually believe that these steps just might work in my favor. Steps one through three geared me up to have enough willingness to tackle Step Four. In Step One, I was honest with myself and able to admit that I couldn't drink like a normal person because I was an alcoholic.

Step Two was fairly easy because I have always believed in a power greater than myself.

Step Three was critical (and became my favorite) because I felt a weight lifted off my shoulders almost instantly. Turning my will and my life over to the care of God helped me to stop trying to control everything in my life. I was then able to do things that I couldn't do before.

For example, Step Four is a step I couldn't have done by myself. I needed God's help and direction to acknowledge my resentments, but more importantly, God helped me realize the part I played in my resentments.

This was surprisingly refreshing, to be able to look at what I could've done differently, and to understand that the pain and anger I held in—for years—was a choice. I was too stubborn to let my anger go, so I held it in, and that resentment was one of the things that fueled my drinking. Step Four can (and will) be extremely difficult without believing in a power greater than yourself.

It is also my recommendation to let God help you through Step Four by placing your will and your life over to His care. This will not only help you to tackle one of the most critical steps, but this will also help you to release anger you thought you could never let go of.

The Turning Point

When I let go of unnecessary anger from holding on to my resentments, I was able to feel pain leave my heart, and old wounds began to heal.

(Hebrews 6:20-11)

*Everything you do in your journey
of self-improvement, including serving
others in love, matters to God.
He wants you to be diligent in meeting
others' needs as well as managing your own.*

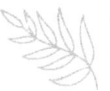 # MY CHARACTER DEFECTS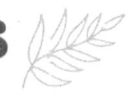

Step Six, and Step Seven helped me to reflect.

I became honest with myself, to point out my defects.

Is this really me? I had to double check.

After getting my sponsor's feedback, I was able to accept.

I have a lot of flaws and they'll be stuck with me for life.

Through God's will, and God's plan, I can learn to use them right.

My shortcomings became principles;

I'm filled with love and no more hate.

I went from loneliness to fellowship,

and my fear transformed to faith.

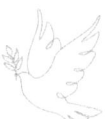

I was able to escape. I was blind but now I see!

When I gave it all to God, He broke the chains and set me free.

My old patterns became my light;

now I feel more useful than before.

I've been moving towards completion, and now I feel restored.

I couldn't ask for more; now God builds with me.

When I gave my life to God, He finally set me free.

My character defects will be stuck with me for life.

Through God's will, and God's plan, I'm learning to use them right.

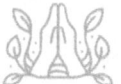 # FROM ME TO YOU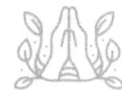

Step Six and Step Seven led me back to what I learned in Step One, which was honesty. Six and Seven allowed me to look in the mirror and point out my character defects and flaws. Being my own critic and using the AA Big Book's outline to embrace and correct my flaws and character defects wasn't an easy task. It wasn't easy because I know myself better than anyone, except God.

Honesty was crucial, if I wanted to move forward as a better human being by accepting that I had a lot of wrinkles that needed to be ironed out. My sponsor helped me to embrace my character defects. He purchased a book for me called "Drop the Rock." Drop the Rock is incredible, and focuses on steps six and seven, removing character defects.

As soon as I read the introduction, I was captivated by what this book had to offer. There was a story about a woman named Mary who was swimming in the water trying to catch up to a boat with her friends and make it to safety. Something kept taking Mary underwater and no matter how hard she tried to swim towards the boat, she felt like she would never catch up, and ultimately drown. Mary's friends were screaming for her to drop the rock, but she didn't understand what they meant. Mary finally understood when she was going down for the third time: this thing around her neck was why she kept sinking when she really wanted to catch the boat! This thing was the "rock" they were all shouting about: resentments, fear, dishonesty, self-pity, intolerance, and anger were just some of the elements her rock was made of. Mary prayed for God to help get rid of the rock, and she caught up to her friends on the boat and made it to safety.

This parable with Mary opened my eyes and allowed me to drop my own rock. I learned that I would continue to drown in my own flaws and character defects if I didn't learn to correct them. In recovery, I learned that we try to take the opposite of our character defects and shortcomings and turn them into principles.

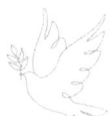

For example, we work to change fear into faith, hate into love, egotism into humility, anxiety and worry into serenity, complacency into action, denial into acceptance, jealousy into trust, fantasy into reality, selfishness into service, resentment into forgiveness, judgmentalism into tolerance, despair into hope, self-hate into respect, and loneliness into fellowship.

Learning this allowed me to embrace my character defects and shortcomings because I understood that I could use the opposite of my flaws as guiding principles.

The Turning Point

When I humbled myself enough to identify my character defects, I was able to transform my flaws into principles.

— • • • —

(Proverbs 11:2-2)

When pride comes, then comes disgrace,
but with humility comes wisdom.

— • • • —

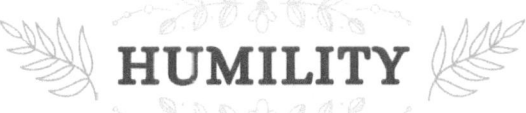

HUMILITY

To find the avenue to freedom, I had to change my attitude.

I became thankful for the small things; now I walk with gratitude.

My spirit was set free, and now my life has stability.

Everything changed when I embraced humility.

God's voice became louder, and now I have brighter days.

God told me to follow his blueprint and the signs along the way.

Being humble is a lifestyle, and that's the path to God.

He wants to push us towards our purpose,

so he trains us for the job.

Today, I'm more patient, and I can feel the shift.

My light from God shines on others, and I appreciate the gift.

Becoming humble changed my life and my blessings have increased.

The dark cloud has been removed; I feel serenity and peace.

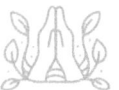 ## FROM ME TO YOU

Humility was something I had to have within me before I could really embrace the twelve steps and become a member of the AA community and fellowship. Step One was extremely difficult, because I never wanted to be labeled as an alcoholic. I thought I was above being labeled as a drunk, an alcoholic, or a person who wasn't able to drink like normal people.

Admitting—to even myself—that I was an alcoholic took way longer than it should have. When I finally hit my bottom and was trapped in the darkest moments of life's journey, I gave in. This was when I became humble.

Humility allowed me to get on my knees and ask God for help. Humility allowed me to stare in the mirror and accept the fact that I could see an alcoholic staring back at me. Humility gave me the strength to be honest with myself. Without humbling myself, I wouldn't have seen any part that I played in my resentments. Without humility, my ego wouldn't have allowed me to address my character defects or make amends.

Today I'm humble enough to believe and understand that my will and my life have been turned over to the care of God. Humility has taught me that I must give away what was given to me freely. Moving forward, I will help other alcoholics to embrace humility, and to find peace and serenity.

The Turning Point

I learned that humility is more than becoming selfless and displaying dignity for a better world. Humility is a lifestyle.

(Romans 12:10)

Be devoted to one another in love.
Honor one another above yourselves.

LIVING WITH OTHERS

I made a list of those I've harmed, and I was willing to make amends.

When I first started the process, I didn't know how it would end.

I had to be objective and keep an open mind.

I had to bury my resentments, and that took a lot of time.

Now that my heart was free, I could see where I went wrong.

I lived with anger, pain, and fear inside of me too long.

When I finally made my list, I had a sense of closure.

A weight was lifted off my shoulders, and it was easy to stay sober.

God's been guiding all my steps, making sure that I don't stumble.

God brought me peace and serenity,

and that helps me to stay humble.

Holding on to grudges is not how I want to live.

It's important I make amends, and learn how to forgive.

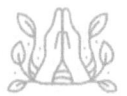 # FROM ME TO YOU

Step Nine was a very important step in my recovery. On Step Nine, I had to try to make amends with anyone I held a resentment towards. I also had to make amends with any place or institution I had resentment against. Being able to find forgiveness in my heart—and more importantly, see the part that I played in my resentments—allowed me to finally have closure.

A fire was burning on the inside of my heart for years, and the flames and smoke that consumed my insides left me in a world of pain. When I finally made amends and forgave everyone and every place (or institution), the pain evaporated almost instantly. It was like a fire truck had finally arrived to put out the flames that had been burning inside of me for years! The fire was put out and the smoke was cleared.

This new feeling of peace and serenity began to engulf my spirit. I felt so good and so free and my anger turned into happiness. I remember thinking to myself: AA really works! The twelve steps can—and will—set you free, if you work them.

I know that without God's help (and letting it be Thy will, and not mine) Step Nine wouldn't have been possible. With that in mind, I'm grateful to have found the power and gifts that the AA Big Book revealed to me. Without God and that book, I don't think I ever would've made my amends.

The Turning Point

When I was able to accept that I played a part in all the built up anger that I'd been holding on to from being resentful, I was able to find the roadmap to finally make my amends.

- - -

(James 5:16)

Therefore, confess your sins to each other and pray for each other so that you may be healed. The prayer of a righteous person is powerful and effective.

- - -

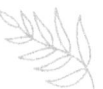 # MAKING MY AMENDS

Resentment and pain caused me years of confusion.
Just recently, I realized that it was all an illusion.
AA and my sponsor helped me make a conclusion.
My relationship with you didn't have to be ruined.
All the resentment I held for years: my heart froze.

Our relationship could've been repaired, but my heart was too cold.

Today, I wrote you this poem to let you know

that our chapter is not closed.

Forgiveness has blossomed in my heart, and I water your rose.

I water your rose, and I give it sunlight.

This is a part of my amends, so this has to be done right.

Moving forward, I want to be a father and son.

No more distance! No more pain! Just laughter and fun.

I apologize for being so stubborn.

The man who helped create me: I didn't know how to love him.

It took for God to call you home for me to shed a tear.

It took for me to make amends to finally face my fears.

I love you with all my heart, and I wish that you were here.

I see you watching over me when the red bird is near.

God speaks through nature, signs, and people.

God can help both of us heal. This can be our sequel.

This time we can do it right.

This time we can let the past be the past and live a better life.

Dad, you're forever in my heart, from now until the end.

I love you Dad! Please forgive me. These are my amends.

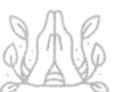 ## FROM ME TO YOU

For as long as I can remember, I've held resentment towards my father. He left me when I was just several months old. He gave me his name and then just disappeared and left me fatherless.

Growing up as a child, I felt so angry because of my abandonment issues. I felt unloved and alone. For years I would express how much I hated my father. I even said that if he died, I wouldn't attend his funeral.

My hatred was fueled by my resentment that I held in for years. I talked to my father face-to-face only five times in my whole life, and I always felt disconnected and disturbed. My anger wouldn't allow me to trust him or learn to love him. On June 12, 2022, my father passed away a week before Father's Day—my older sister called me on my way to work with the news. I thought that I wouldn't care, or that I wouldn't be affected by his death...but I was wrong.

I couldn't work. I couldn't think. I felt like I couldn't breathe. The man who I barely knew was gone, and I didn't want him to be. I missed him and I realized that my anger stemmed from a buried pain, because deep down inside...I loved him.

When my dad died, my drinking took off like a rocket. I didn't want to feel the pain of losing him and not being able to have closure from all the pain and resentment I was still carrying. My dad was a drug addict and an alcoholic who abandoned me: this is why I felt resentful towards him. I discovered that while doing Step Four.

I also discovered the part I played while doing my columns: I was also an alcoholic, just like my father. I also abandoned my children when I went to prison, and took them through the same pain I experienced as a child.

How could I hold onto resentment towards my father when I had done the same things he had? This made me feel even more guilty after his death because I ignored his calls and his messages, and now he was gone.

How would I release this pain? How could I make amends with my father? These were questions I was asking myself. I needed a way to be free from my resentment and pain. My sponsor helped me with my resentment and amends for my father; he recommended that I write my father a letter.

After writing my father a poem, I felt at peace. I believe he has found peace in heaven as well.

The Turning Point

When I made amends for all my resentments, a heavy weight was lifted off my shoulders. My anger disappeared, and I finally felt free from the pain that lived inside of me for years.

Forgiveness is a powerful tool that has brought me peace and serenity.

• • •

(Proverbs 3:5-6)

Trust in the Lord with all your heart, and do not lean on your own understanding. In all your ways acknowledge him, and he will make straight paths. Ultimately, being a better person means putting our trust in God and seeking his guidance in all aspects of our lives.

• • •

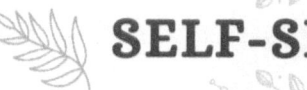# SELF-SEARCHING

I take my inventory daily, and when I'm wrong...I admit it.

This helps me to stay humble, and this keeps me on my pivot.

Can I stay sober? I constantly ask myself this question.

How can I prevent a relapse? It can happen at any second.

I ask myself these questions because it helps me to check my pride.

Being cocky can become detrimental,

and I can stumble in my stride.

I have to stay aware of all the roadblocks and

the snares along the way.

Becoming sober wasn't easy, but this is where I want to stay.

Self-searching is a regular habit, and Step Ten is a daily practice.

Checking my inventory is critical, and I'm constantly taking action.

Emotional hangovers happen often,

but I refuse to let pain and fear win.

I'll regroup then I'll reset, and then it's back to Step Ten.

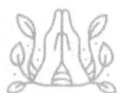# FROM ME TO YOU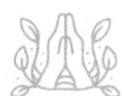

Step Ten is a powerful tool that I was able to add to my tool belt. Anytime I'm feeling unbalanced and off the beam, I take my personal inventory. Step Ten keeps me humble, honest, and focused.

In the past, it was difficult for me to admit when I was wrong. I would fight tooth and nail to stand on my opinion and what I thought was right. Now, I practice Step Ten, and when I'm wrong I won't hesitate to admit it. When I'm feeling resentful, I'll quickly calm myself to get rid of anger. If there's a situation where I need to apologize and make amends, I'll do it!

Emotional hangovers are something that I don't have to experience when I'm continuing to take my personal inventory. It's like I'm constantly checking the air in my tires, the oil levels, my brakes, and the engine light. This step keeps me tuned up and my daily ride is smooth.

When I retire at night, I constructively review my day. Was I resentful, selfish, dishonest, or afraid? Do I owe anyone an apology? Have I kept something to myself that should be discussed with another person at once? This ritual allows me to close my eyes after my prayer, feeling like I gave my all to be the best version of myself for that day.

The Turning Point

Step Ten has become a daily practice. This step taught me how important it is to constantly check my personal inventory. When I'm wrong, I must admit it. Self-searching every day allows me to stay humble and less prideful.

This has become a powerful tool for examining my character and who I am as a person. Step Ten constantly helps me to tighten up any loose screws within myself.

. . .

(Psalms 119:27)

Make me understand the way of your precepts,
and I will meditate on your wondrous works.

. . .

 # PRAYER AND MEDITATION

Praying to God is so powerful, and that's how I stay connected.
When I'm lost, God takes my hand and makes sure I'm redirected.
God gives me grace and mercy
—that's why I'm never feeling hopeless.
Through prayer and meditation, I taught myself to focus.
I learned to use my spiritual eyes
and I learned to use my spiritual ears.
I was blind, but now I see. I was deaf, but now I hear.
Only God knows the chapter that my purpose was written in.

To live out God's will for my life, I have to stay disciplined.

I have to stay humble, and I must remain grateful.

That's why I'll never stop praying, because I must remain faithful.

I'm in the passenger seat and God's behind the wheel.

God has the GPS for my life, so I let it be Thy will.

My seatbelt is on and I'm ready for the ride!

My ego has disappeared, and I let go of my pride.

It's God's will, not mine—that's what I had to understand.

Now that I've submitted, God can carry out his plan.

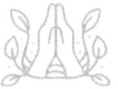 FROM ME TO YOU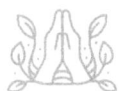

Prayer and meditation have become a part of my everyday ritual. After finishing Step Three I felt at peace because for the first time in my life I was able to believe and understand that God's will was what would bring me serenity. My spiritual eyes were finally opened, and I could see that God had a bigger plan for my life than I could ever imagine.

I buckled up my seatbelt and accepted my role in the passenger seat. God has the GPS towards my purpose and the plans he has for my life; all he wants me to do is to stay connected to His will, not mine.

How do I stay connected? This was what I learned in Step Eleven: how to improve my conscious contact with God as I understood Him. Through prayer and meditation, I am able to stay connected to God and His will for my life.

This feeling of having a constant connection with God almighty has been powerful, beautiful, peaceful, and refreshing. I have become so accustomed to praying and meditating that I lose count of how many times I do it on a daily basis. It's more than a routine—it's a way of life. God wants to build with me. That alone makes my heart smile and gives me hope for a bright future filled with purpose and better days ahead.

The Turning Point

Prayer and meditation have allowed me to have conscious contact with God. Step Eleven became my blueprint to use my spiritual eyes and ears, to see and hear God's plans for my life. Through prayer and meditation, I am able to follow the path that He has set towards my purpose, and the plans He has for my life.

— · · · —

(1 Peter 1:13)

Therefore, with minds that are alert and fully sober, set your hope on grace to be brought to you when Jesus Christ is revealed at His coming.

— · · · —

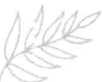

MY SPIRITUAL AWAKENING

The spiritual awakening is something I was chasing.

I knew I wouldn't capture it overnight, so I had to practice patience.

I wanted peace and serenity. I wanted my pain and fear to be gone.

I have been dreaming about these moments;

I prayed and prayed for so long!

I knew it wouldn't fall into my lap and that I had to do the work.

I took the twelve steps seriously, and that's what started my rebirth.

In Step One I was honest, and then in Step Three I submitted.

After Step Four I was less angry and became more committed.

Step Six and Step Seven helped me to see the man in the mirror.

Step Nine taught me forgiveness, and my vision became clear.

Step Ten became a daily practice to examine my motives.

Step Eleven is critical, and it helps me to focus.

When I pray and meditate,

that strengthens my connection with God.

God has the GPS for my life, so I never feel lost.

God's purpose for my life is to uplift my sisters and brothers.

I have to give away what I have, and share it with others.

I had a spiritual awakening, as a result of these steps.

Now I will carry this message to other alcoholics,

until my very last breath.

 # FROM ME TO YOU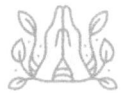

The spiritual awakening is not something that I captured after completing Step Twelve; I felt it in spurts. After completing Step One and being honest about being an alcoholic, I felt better in my spirit. After completing Step Three, and turning my will and my life over to the care of God, I felt my spirit waking up instantly. Steps four through nine is when I realized that my spirit was becoming stronger and fully awake. I felt less angry after completing Step Four. I was able to accept and correct my flaws on steps six and seven. Step Nine soothed my soul after making amends. By the time I got to Step Eleven, I was eager to keep the fire burning in my spirit through prayer and meditation. God had awakened my spirit and was strengthening my heart and soul for Step Twelve and beyond.

Today, I understand that to keep my spirit awake I have to continue to carry out God's message to other alcoholics. The process of having a spiritual awakening and keeping my soul alive includes constantly taking action towards helping others by giving away what was freely given to me.

The Turning Point

To stay awake spiritually, I have to continue to do God's will, not mine. I will continue to carry the message to other alcoholics.

• • •

(Philippians 2:2)

Complete my joy by being of the same mind,
having the same love, being in full accord
and of one mind.

• • •

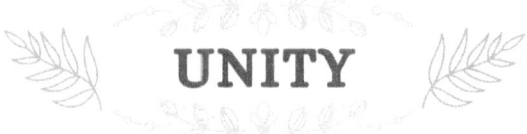

UNITY

Isolation was so lonely and detrimental for my health.

I was an alcoholic in denial—I couldn't get sober by myself.

Unity is priceless; I've found a fellowship and built a bond.

Now, I don't feel alone on this journey that I'm on.

When I attend an AA meeting it's filled with alcoholics just like me.

Through our testimonies, no one is invisible.

We hear each other and we see.

We hear each other's pain, and we wipe each other's tears.
We uplift one another and help calm each other's fears.
God led us here. He brought us through the rainy weather.
Finally, the sun is shining on us,
and we can feel the warmth together.

High Off Life

Finding the fellowship that AA had to offer brought me peace, serenity, strength, togetherness, and happiness. This unity has been a key component to my sobriety and my mental and emotional wellbeing.

• • •

(Ephesians 5:18)

And do not get drunk off wine,
for that is debauchery,
but be filled with the spirit.

• • •

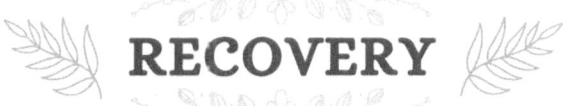

RECOVERY

My recovery is a process that didn't happen overnight.

I went from abusing alcohol to being sober

—I came from the darkness to the light.

My journey is ongoing, and I'll be traveling for life.

Relapses are unexpected, so I keep my routine tight.

I stay in contact with my sponsor because

he helped me beat the odds.

He saved me from the bottle; I was stuck and I was lost.

The bond I built with my sponsor brought me humility and patience.

He led me through the steps, and I had a spiritual awakening.

God used my sponsor to help to set me free.

Being sober is a gift and I embrace recovery.

Now my life is filled with purpose, new meaning,

and understanding.

This was all God's will, and a part of God's planning.

God's purpose for my life is to carry

the twelve step message to others.

I have to give away what I've learned to all my sisters and brothers.

To the alcoholic who still suffers: today can be your day!

Through God's will and God's plan, you'll find a better way.

High Off Life

The road to recovery was a process I couldn't do alone. I needed God, sponsorship, and a strong fellowship. I also had to be more honest with myself than I'd ever been. Lastly, I had to practice humility and willingness. I became grateful for the opportunity to become sober and free. I had to understand that God stepped into my life, and that my will was no longer in effect.

· · ·

(Proverbs 11:25)

A generous person will prosper;
whoever refreshes others will be refreshed.

· · ·

SERVICE

To give freely is unselfish. To help struggling alcoholics is a gift.
Sobriety can make the world a better place,
and we can help to make the shift.
My sponsor helped me; now, it's my turn to help another.
We can give each other hope by staying connected to each other.

Our fellowship will grow, each and every day.

There are millions still in pain, and yearning to be saved.

Take hold of my hand; I'll lead you to the way.

You'll find peace and serenity and that's where you'll want to stay.

You'll be free from pain and fear, and safe from any wreckage.

Then through God's will and God's plan,

you can carry out his message.

Let's help those who are hopeless—we can teach them to be free.

We'll conquer alcoholism together; let's heal the world, you and me.

High Off Life

The greatest gifts I received in sobriety were wisdom, knowledge, and understanding. I was able to internalize what the AA Big Book and twelve steps taught me. I became aware of God's will and His plans for my life. Today, I understand that the gift of sobriety must be given away if I want to keep it. Helping others to find peace, serenity, and freedom through sobriety is how God strengthens our willingness to remain sober ourselves.

• • •

(Proverbs 24:26)

An honest answer is like a kiss on the lips.

• • •

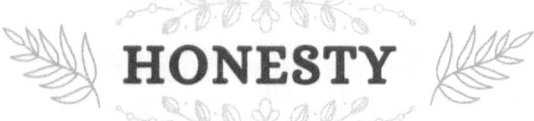

HONESTY

When I'm staring in the mirror, I can't hide from my reflection.

Being truthful with myself leads me in the right direction.

I'm an alcoholic. That took a while to admit.

I was embarrassed to say I was, and it was hard to submit.

When I finally became comfortable accepting all my flaws,

Life became more meaningful, and I started living with a cause.

I could identify my pain and I finally faced my fears.

Drinking was never the solution, but I thought it was for years.

Today I use the twelve steps to help me stay aligned.

Being honest helped me to transform, and that took a lot of time.

Transparency with myself unlocked the doors—that was the key.

Dishonesty kept me shackled, until the truth set me free.

High Off Life

I learned that by being completely honest with myself, I could continue to grow and become a better human being. Living a lie would weaken my connection with God, and living life being dishonest blocks the connection to my purpose and God's plans for my life. Honesty taught me that the truth will set you free.

(Matthew 5:8)
Blessed are the pure in heart,
for they shall see God.

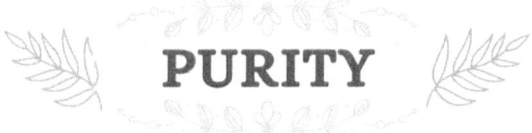

PURITY

My vision is clear and now I can see God's plan.

God wants to use me as a vessel, and now I understand.

His purpose for my life is to spread love and bring peace.

No more worries. No more fear. Everything shall cease.

Faith will fill our hearts; in a higher power, we shall believe.

If you submit your life to God, then anything can be achieved.

Our life is in His hands; God wants to build with us.

Do you believe it? Do you have faith? All you have to do is trust.

Remain pure in our hearts, and God will give us room to grow.

If you pray and meditate, then you already know.

When we were born, God had plans for every boy and every girl.

There's a purpose for all of us and we shall share it with the world.

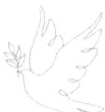

High Off Life

When my heart became pure I felt alive in my soul. God's presence became stronger in my life, and my spiritual eyes were now open.

· · ·

(1 Corinthians 10:24)

No one should seek their own good,
but the good of others.

· · ·

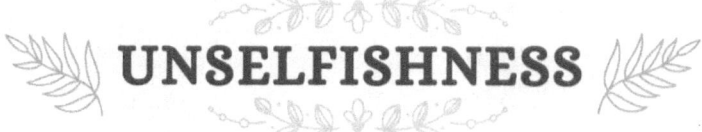

UNSELFISHNESS

I'm living my life to help others—I'm not focused on myself.
Bringing smiles to those with frowns means
more than gaining wealth.
The world is plagued with hate, that's why I want to spread my love.
To anyone that's feeling pain, I'll embrace you with a hug.
Kindness and compassion are what I'm here to share.
My heart is open to the world to let you know I care.
Do you need someone to talk to? I'm here to listen, if you do.

Your pain is my pain. Please, let me help you see it through.

Grab my hand and let me lead you to the place where I found peace.

God has a place where your pain will instantly decrease.

Give your life to God, and put others before yourself.

Become selfless, and if someone's struggling,

extend your hand and offer help.

High Off Life

Becoming selfless and putting others before myself has transformed my spirit, and I feel purposeful in God's plans for my life. Love your neighbor as you love yourself. Do more for others than you do for yourself. This way of life is so rewarding, and has brought me closer to God than I've ever been.

(1 Corinthians 13:4-8)

Love is patient, love is kind. It does not envy,
it does not boast, it is not proud. It does not
dishonor others, it is not self-seeking, it is not
easily angered, it keeps no records of wrongs.
Love does not delight in evil but rejoices with the
truth. It always protects, it always trusts, always
hopes, always perseveres. Love never fails.

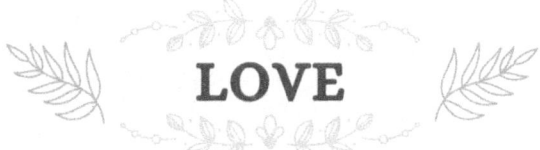

LOVE

She has the most beautiful smile, and her heart seems so pure.

I've heard her share her testimony in AA meetings,

but I'm yearning to hear more.

This woman seems so special, and I can tell she's been restored.

When I see her, her light is shining from the ceiling to the floor.

She's been sober for over two years, and that's not an easy task.

I can tell that she submitted her will to God

—I don't even have to ask.

We will meet many people in this lifetime,

and they'll give us different vibes.

Every time I hugged this woman, she made me feel alive.

There's something about her...it's like her presence is a gift.

When she enters the room, positivity flows, and I can feel the shift.

I'm grateful that I met her. I can't wait to get to know her better.

She is one of those special people that I'd like to know forever.

High Off Life

Love is one of God's greatest gifts. Having a bond and a meaningful
friendship with a person you can trust and depend on is priceless.

— • • • —

(1 Peter 5:8)

Be sober-minded; be watchful. Your adversary
the devil prowls around like a roaring lion,
seeking someone to devour.

— • • • —

 # KEEP COMING BACK

Today, I'm grateful to be nine months clean.

Waking up sober still feels like a dream.

God showed me grace when he led me to AA.

Now I'm high off life, and this is where I want to stay.

I found peace and serenity, and my life has been restored.

AA is my home: I love walking through those doors!

On my drive back home, I'm always grateful for the meetings.

Your testimonies give me hope, and I appreciate your greetings.

The meetings are filled with love and alcoholics just like me.

I found purpose in the fellowship; I was blind but now I see.

I don't have to isolate and do this by myself.

That's why I keep coming back, because these meetings really help.

Where do I see myself in three months? I'll be sober and full of faith.

I'll be standing at the podium...

receiving my chip and getting some cake.

High Off Life

When I reached nine months of sobriety, it felt like nine years to me. For the first time in my life, I felt so alive and free! I was mesmerized at how much my life had changed by just giving my life to God and working the twelve steps. I was headed towards my year mark, and the feeling was priceless. I remember saying to myself: *keep coming back; it works if you work it!*

(1 Peter 4:7)

The end of all things is at hand;
therefore, be self-controlled and sober-minded
for the sake of your prayers.

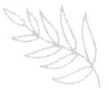 # ONE DAY AT A TIME

One day at a time. Twenty four hours are here, and then it's over.

One day at a time. I pray to God to keep me sober.

One day at a time. I have to stick to my routine.

One day at a time. Today's meeting kept me clean.

One day at a time. I keep my sobriety in a vice grip.

One day at a time. My fellowship is priceless.

One day at a time. Today's another day to go conquer.

One day at a time. I won't forget to call my sponsor.

One day at a time. There's a power greater than myself.

One day at a time. Through God's will, I'll get help.

One day at a time. That's all I have to remember.

One day at a time. If I make it through today, I'm a winner.

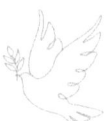

High Off Life

The most important day of your sobriety is the current day. Don't get caught up in how you got sober. Don't become overconfident in how long you've been sober, and don't lose focus by concentrating on the milestones that may be ahead. Stay in the present. Focus on the day at hand and everything will take care of itself. One day at a time. Keep it simple.

• • •

(Psalms 34:18)

The Lord is close to the broken-hearted
and saves those who are crushed in spirit.

• • •

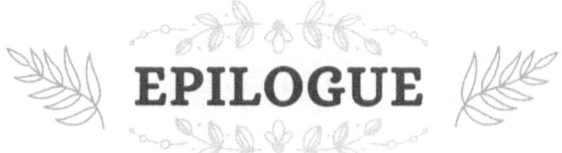

EPILOGUE

In the past, I was able to drink like a normal person. Drinking alcohol was something I was able to do socially and have a good time. Suddenly, my life became overwhelming, and filled with pain, and my drinking took a turn for the worse.

My drinking went from zero to ten and became a crutch to help ease all the pain, fear, and trauma that I was dealing with.

I started drinking large amounts of alcohol every day, all day. This ritual of abusive drinking led me to dislike the man in the mirror. Who was this person? Who had I become? The answer was staring me in the face as I held a bottle of liquor in my hand while staring at my reflection. Am I an alcoholic? I asked myself. Of course I am!

This reality was extremely difficult for me to accept. I never thought I would fall into the category of being a person who couldn't control how much alcohol they consumed. With the hard part (being honest with myself) out of the way, what was I going to do next?

The only solution I could think of was to ask God to release me of my bondage to alcohol. I took action, got down on my knees, and asked God to save me from my addiction. God heard my prayers, and before I could continue killing myself...God blessed me with a sponsor.

My sponsor was a gift from God.

Without God sending my sponsor into my life to save me, I can't imagine where I'd be today.

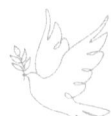

My sponsor led me down the road to recovery by introducing me to AA and The Big Book. He took me through the twelve steps; the process of internalizing each step and thoroughly completing them, one by one, was life changing. For the first time in my life, I felt free as a bird!

It was as if I grew wings and was soaring through the sky. This was a spiritual experience, and a spiritual awakening.

With my sponsor's help, I found myself closer to God than I'd ever been. All my worries, my pain, and fears were gone. My light began to shine, and I was ready to carry out God's mission by giving away what was given to me. It was my turn to help someone who was struggling like I was. It was my turn to carry out the message of sobriety, and all the promises that AA had to offer.

Today, I can say with my chest that I'm an alcoholic. This honesty and transparency has brought me out of the darkness into the light!

To the alcoholic who still suffers, I want you to know that there is light at the end of the tunnel. There is relief for the pain that you may be feeling at the moment. Your fears, your worries, and all life's obstacles can be overcome. All you need to do is to have the willingness and faith to believe that there is a power greater than yourself. If you open your mind, heart, and soul to this power, I guarantee you will not regret doing so.

This will open the gates of freedom, peace, and serenity. This will allow you to turn your will and your life over to the care of God, as you understand him. God's plan for our life is the key to sobriety, spiritual freedom, happiness, and purpose.

High Off Life

Today is a great day to be sober!

Available by Lewis Burt

I STILL CAN'T BREATHE
400 YEARS LATER

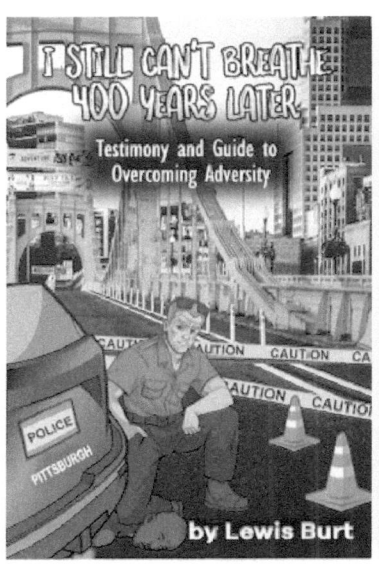

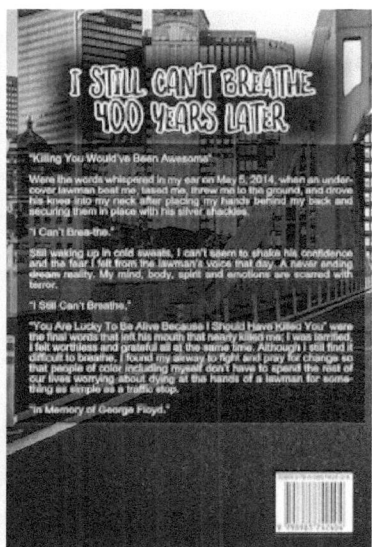

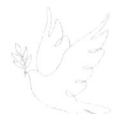

SAVE THE BLACK MAN
BLESSINGS IN DISGUISE

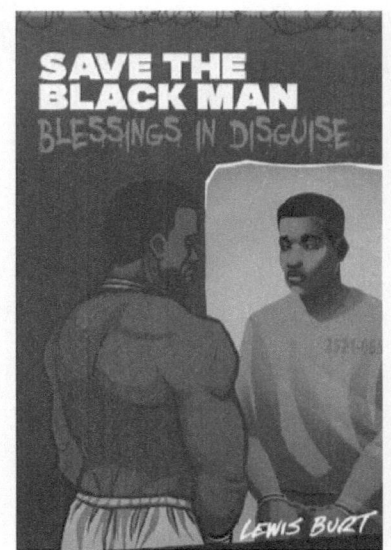
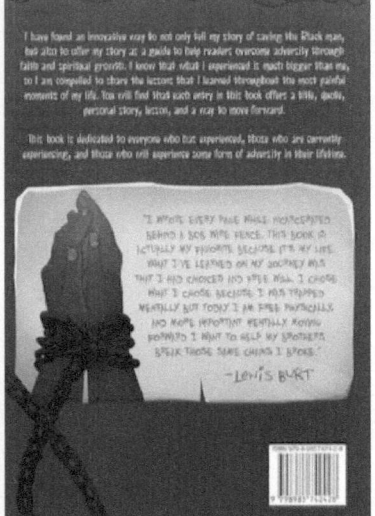

YOUR PRESIDENT KILLED AMERICA
NEW WORLD ORDER

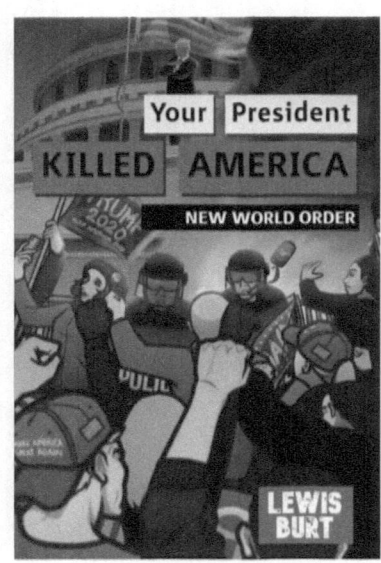
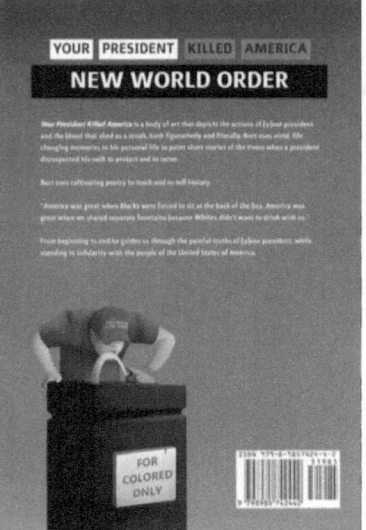

www.ingramcontent.com/pod-product-compliance
Lightning Source LLC
Chambersburg PA
CBHW020340130626
46549CB00003B/1233